I0703345

Fatty liver disease

Guide on how to manage Fatty liver disease with some essential good food and fruit

Dr Joe smith

Contents

chapter1

introduction to fatty liver disease diet

Fatty liver disease   also known as hepatic steatosis, is a condition in which fat accumulates in the liver cells. This buildup of fat can lead to inflammation and damage to the liver, which is responsible for important functions such as detoxifying the blood, storing energy, and producing bile. There are two main types of fatty liver disease: non-alcoholic fatty liver disease (NAFLD) and alcoholic fatty liver disease (AFLD). NAFLD is the most common form and is usually caused by factors such as obesity, insulin resistance, and high levels of fats in the blood. AFLD, on the other hand, is caused by managing Fatty liver disease with some essential good food and fruit alcohol consumption and is often seen in people who consume large amounts of alcohol on a regular basis. A key factor in managing and treating fatty liver disease is a healthy diet. The right diet can help reduce the amount of fat in the liver and prevent further damage. In this article, we will discuss the important components of a fatty liver disease diet and provide tips for making healthy dietary changes. Limiting Calories and Weight Loss For those who are overweight or obese, the first step in managing fatty liver disease is to lose weight. Excess weight, especially around the waist, is a significant risk factor for developing NAFLD. In fact, studies have shown that losing 7-10% of body weight can significantly improve liver function and reduce the amount of fat in the liver. The key to weight loss is creating a calorie deficit, which means burning more calories than you consume. A healthy rate of weight loss is 1-2 pounds per week, so it is important to be patient and consistent with your efforts. It is also important to note that fad or crash diets are not recommended for individuals with fatty liver disease. These types of diets may lead to rapid weight loss, but they are not sustainable and can be harmful to overall health. Instead, focus on making gradual and sustainable dietary changes that will support long-term weight loss and management. Healthy Carbohydrates Carbohydrates are an essential source of energy for the body, but not all carbohydrates are created equal. When it comes to managing fatty liver disease, it is important to focus on consuming healthy carbohydrates that are high in fiber and low in added sugars. Fiber is an important nutrient for individuals with fatty liver disease as it helps slow down the absorption of sugar and can help improve insulin resistance. Insulin resistance is a condition in which the body does not effectively use insulin, a hormone that helps transport sugar from the blood into the cells to be used for energy. High levels of sugar in the blood can contribute to the development and progression of fatty liver disease. Some healthy sources of carbohydrates to include in a fatty liver disease diet include whole grains, fruits, vegetables, and legumes. These foods are not only high in fiber, but they also contain important vitamins and minerals that can help support overall health. Limiting processed and refined carbohydrates such as white bread, white rice, and sugary snacks and drinks is important for managing fatty liver disease. These foods are typically high in added sugars and lack essential nutrients, which can contribute to weight gain and further liver damage. Protein Protein is an important nutrient for maintaining and repairing body tissues, including the liver. Adequate protein intake is essential for individuals with fatty liver disease as it can help prevent muscle loss and support weight loss efforts.

When choosing protein sources, it is important to opt for lean options such as skinless chicken, fish, beans, and legumes. Avoiding fatty cuts of meat and processed meats is important as they can contribute to weight gain and further liver damage. Moderate Alcohol Consumption For individuals with AFLD, avoiding or limiting alcohol consumption is crucial for managing fatty liver disease. Alcohol is toxic to liver cells and can lead to inflammation and scarring, making it difficult for the liver to function properly. If you have been diagnosed with AFLD, it is important to consult with a healthcare professional about your alcohol consumption. In general, it is recommended to have no more than one drink per day for women and two drinks per day for men. It is also important to note that alcohol should not be consumed during pregnancy. Other Dietary Considerations Aside from limiting certain foods and managing weight, there are other dietary considerations that can help support liver health for individuals with fatty liver disease. Incorporating healthy fats, such as avocados, nuts, and fatty fish, into the diet can provide important nutrients and may help improve insulin sensitivity. Choosing low-glycemic index (GI) foods can also be beneficial for individuals with fatty liver disease. The glycemic index is a system that ranks foods based on how much they increase blood sugar levels. Foods with a high GI, such as white bread and sugary snacks, can cause a spike in blood sugar levels, which is not ideal for managing fatty liver disease. Low-GI foods, such as whole grains, nuts, and beans, are digested more slowly, leading to a more gradual rise in blood sugar levels. Lastly, staying well-hydrated is important for liver health. Drinking enough water can help flush out toxins from the body and support overall liver function. In Conclusion A healthy diet is a crucial component of managing and treating fatty liver disease. By making dietary changes such as limiting calories, focusing on healthy carbohydrates and protein sources, and avoiding or limiting alcohol consumption, individuals with fatty liver disease can improve their liver health and prevent further damage. It is important to consult with a healthcare professional and registered dietitian to create a personalized dietary plan that meets your individual needs and goals. With the right diet and lifestyle changes, fatty liver disease can be managed and future complications can be prevented.

Chapter2

Essential Foods for Managing Fatty Liver Disease

The good news is that fatty liver disease is largely reversible through diet and lifestyle changes. One of the most effective ways to manage and prevent this condition is by consuming a healthy and balanced diet. In this article, we will discuss some of the essential foods that have been shown to be beneficial for managing fatty liver disease. 1. Fruits and Vegetables Fruits and vegetables are important for managing any type of health condition, and fatty liver disease is no exception. These nutritious foods are packed with vitamins, minerals, antioxidants, and fiber, making them essential for maintaining a healthy liver. A diet rich in fruits and vegetables has been shown to reduce the risk of fatty liver disease, as well as improving liver function in those who already have the condition. Some of the best fruits and vegetables for managing fatty liver disease include leafy greens such as spinach and kale, brightly colored berries, cruciferous vegetables like broccoli and cauliflower, and citrus fruits like oranges and grapefruits. These foods are not only low in calories and rich in essential nutrients, but they also possess anti-inflammatory properties that can help reduce liver inflammation, a common symptom of fatty liver disease. 2. Whole Grains Whole grains are another essential food for managing fatty liver disease. Unlike refined grains, which have been stripped of their fiber and nutrients, whole grains still contain the bran and germ, making them a good source of fiber, vitamins, and minerals. These nutrients are essential for maintaining liver health and reducing the risk of fatty liver disease. Whole grains, such as oats, quinoa, brown rice, and whole wheat, are also low in glycemic index, which means they have a slower effect on blood sugar levels. This is important for managing fatty liver disease, as high blood sugar levels can increase the risk of liver damage. Consuming whole grains as part of a balanced diet can also help with weight management, as they can help you feel fuller for longer and reduce cravings for unhealthy foods. 3. Lean Protein Protein is an essential nutrient for overall health, and it is particularly important for managing fatty liver disease. However, not all protein sources are created equal. It is important to choose lean protein sources, such as chicken, fish, and tofu, as they are low in unhealthy fats and can help reduce liver fat accumulation. Protein also plays a crucial role in repairing and regenerating liver cells, which is important for those with fatty liver disease. Additionally, consuming lean protein sources can help with weight loss and weight management, which is beneficial for those with fatty liver disease as excess weight is a major risk factor for this condition. 4. Healthy Fats Contrary to popular belief, not all fats are bad for you. In fact, some types of fat are essential for maintaining a healthy liver. Healthy fats, such as monounsaturated and polyunsaturated fats found in foods like avocados, olive oil, and fatty fish, have been shown to improve liver health and reduce the risk of fatty liver disease. These fats are also important for reducing inflammation in the body, which is a common symptom of fatty liver disease. However, it is important to consume healthy fats in moderation, as they are still high in calories. Aim for a balance of healthy fats, lean protein, and complex carbohydrates in your diet to maintain a healthy liver. 5. Green Tea Green tea has been touted for its numerous health benefits, and its effects on liver health are no exception. This popular beverage is rich in antioxidants, especially a compound called catechin, which has been shown to have anti-inflammatory effects on the liver. In addition, studies have found that green tea can reduce liver fat and improve liver function in those with fatty liver disease. To reap the potential liver-protecting benefits of green tea, aim for 2-3 cups a day. You can also add lemon or honey to your tea for added flavor and potential detoxifying properties. 6. Nuts and Seeds Nuts and seeds are a great source of healthy fats, fiber, and protein, making them a beneficial food for managing fatty liver disease. Some studies have found that consuming nuts, such as almonds and walnuts, can help reduce liver fat and improve liver function in those with this condition. However, it is important to consume nuts and seeds in moderation, as they are high in calories. A small handful a day is enough to reap their nutritional benefits without overdoing it. 7. Probiotic Foods Probiotics, also known as good bacteria, have been shown to have a positive effect on liver health. These beneficial bacteria can be found in fermented foods such as yogurt, kefir, sauerkraut, and kimchi. Probiotic foods help maintain a healthy gut microbiome, which is essential for overall health and can play a role in reducing liver inflammation. In addition, probiotics may also help improve insulin resistance, a common risk factor for fatty liver disease. Aim to incorporate these foods into your diet regularly for optimal liver health. 8. Lean Red Meat While consuming too much red meat can be harmful to overall health, lean cuts of red meat, such as beef, lamb, and pork, can be beneficial for managing fatty liver disease. Red meat is a good source of iron, zinc, and B vitamins, which are important for maintaining liver function. However, it is important to consume red meat in moderation and opt for lean cuts to avoid consuming excessive unhealthy fats. Aim for no more than 2-3 servings of red meat per week and balance it with other sources of lean protein. 9. Coffee While coffee is not typically considered a "health food," studies have found that moderate coffee consumption may have a protective effect on liver health. Coffee contains compounds that have anti-inflammatory and antioxidant properties, which can help reduce liver inflammation and protect against fatty liver disease. However, it is important to consume coffee in moderation, as excessive caffeine intake can have negative effects on overall health. Aim for no more than 2-3 cups of coffee per day. 10. Water Lastly, staying hydrated by drinking enough water is crucial for managing fatty liver disease. Water helps flush out toxins and waste products from the body, including the liver. Dehydration can also lead to increased liver fat accumulation, which is why it is essential to drink plenty of water throughout the day. It is recommended to drink at least 8-10 cups of water per day, but this may vary depending on individual needs. Aim to drink water instead of sugary beverages such as sodas or fruit juices to avoid excess sugar intake, which can contribute to liver fat accumulation.

.

Chapter3

The important of vitamin e in treating fatty liver disease

Fatty liver disease, also known as hepatic steatosis, is a serious condition that occurs when excessive fat builds up in the liver. This can lead to inflammation and damage to the liver, impairing its ability to function properly. While excessive alcohol consumption is a common cause of fatty liver disease, it can also occur in individuals who do not drink alcohol, a condition known as non-alcoholic fatty liver disease (NAFLD). According to the American Liver Foundation, NAFLD affects nearly 100 million people in the United States alone. Fatty liver disease can range in severity from a mild condition, where it may not cause any noticeable symptoms, to a more serious and potentially life-threatening condition known as non-alcoholic steatohepatitis (NASH). NASH is a progressive form of fatty liver disease that involves not only the buildup of fat in the liver, but also inflammation and damage to liver cells. Left untreated, NASH can progress to further liver damage, cirrhosis, and ultimately, liver failure. Thankfully, there are several treatment options available for fatty liver disease, with one of the most promising being the use of vitamin E. Vitamin E is a fat-soluble vitamin that plays a crucial role in maintaining overall health and wellness. It is primarily known for its antioxidant properties, which protect the body from free radicals and oxidative stress. However, recent research has shown that vitamin E also has a significant role in treating fatty liver disease, making it a vital component in the management and prevention of this condition. One of the main reasons why vitamin E is important in treating fatty liver disease is its antioxidant properties. Oxidative stress refers to an imbalance between free radicals, which are highly reactive molecules, and the body's natural antioxidant defenses. Excessive free radicals can cause damage to cells and tissues, leading to inflammation and various diseases, including fatty liver disease. Vitamin E works to neutralize these free radicals and reduce oxidative stress, thereby protecting the liver from damage and preventing the progression of fatty liver disease. Studies have also shown that vitamin E can help reduce inflammation in the liver, a key factor in the development and progression of fatty liver disease. Inflammation is the body's natural response to injury or infection, but chronic inflammation can damage liver cells and promote further scarring and fibrosis in the liver. Vitamin E has been found to inhibit the production of pro-inflammatory cytokines, compounds that play a significant role in the inflammatory process, thus helping to reduce liver inflammation and prevent further damage. Moreover, vitamin E has been shown to have a positive impact on the liver's fat metabolism. A healthy liver absorbs and metabolizes fat, converting it into energy or storing it for later use. In fatty liver disease, this process is impaired, causing fat to accumulate in the liver. Vitamin E has been found to promote fat metabolism in the liver, helping to decrease fat buildup and prevent the progression of fatty liver disease. Apart from its direct effects on the liver, vitamin E also plays a crucial role in managing other conditions that can contribute to fatty liver disease. For example, obesity and diabetes are often associated with fatty liver disease and can worsen its symptoms. As a potent antioxidant, vitamin E can help manage these conditions by reducing inflammation and improving insulin sensitivity, thus indirectly contributing to the treatment of fatty liver disease. The effectiveness of vitamin E in treating fatty liver disease has been supported by multiple studies. In a 2015 study, researchers found that vitamin E supplementation significantly improved liver enzyme levels, a marker of liver function, in individuals with NAFLD. Another study conducted in 2018 found that vitamin E supplementation was effective in reducing liver fat and reverse liver scarring in patients with NASH. These findings suggest that vitamin E supplementation can be a valuable tool in treating and managing fatty liver disease. It is important to note that while vitamin E is an excellent option for treating fatty liver disease, it is not a cure-all solution. Lifestyle changes, such as maintaining a healthy diet and regular exercise, are also crucial in managing and preventing fatty liver disease. Additionally, individuals with fatty liver disease should consult their healthcare provider before starting any vitamin E supplementation, as excessive doses may have adverse effects. , vitamin E plays a vital role in treating fatty liver disease by reducing oxidative stress, inflammation, and improving fat metabolism in the liver. In combination with other lifestyle changes, such as a healthy diet and regular exercise, vitamin E can help prevent and manage fatty liver disease, ultimately leading to better liver function and improved overall health. More research is still needed to fully understand the mechanisms behind vitamin E's effects on fatty liver disease, but current evidence supports its importance as a potential treatment option. By recognizing and utilizing the benefits of vitamin E, we can take a significant step towards combatting this widespread and serious health condition. Moreover, Vitamin E has been shown to improve insulin sensitivity, which is an important factor in the development and progression of NAFLD. Insulin resistance, a condition where the body's cells do not respond properly to insulin, is closely linked to NAFLD. This is because the liver plays a role in breaking down and storing insulin, and when liver function is compromised, it can lead to insulin resistance. By improving insulin sensitivity, Vitamin E can help to prevent the progression of NAFLD and potentially reverse the condition. In addition to its beneficial effects on NAFLD, Vitamin E has been found to have a positive impact on other health conditions that commonly co-occur with this condition. For instance, patients with NAFLD are at a higher risk of developing cardiovascular disease, and Vitamin E has been found to have a protective effect on the cardiovascular system. A 2015 study published in the Journal of Atherosclerosis and Thrombosis found that Vitamin E supplementation was able to improve endothelial function, reduce oxidative stress, and improve lipid profiles in patients with NAFLD. Furthermore,

Vitamin E has also been found to be beneficial in improving non-alcoholic steatohepatitis (NASH), a more severe form of NAFLD. NASH is characterized by liver inflammation and may progress to cirrhosis and liver failure if left untreated. A 2018 study published in the Journal of Hepatology found that Vitamin E supplementation was able to improve liver function and reduce inflammation in patients with NASH. While Vitamin E has shown promising results in treating NAFLD, it is essential to note that it should not be used as a standalone treatment. Lifestyle changes, such as maintaining a healthy weight, following a balanced diet, and incorporating regular exercise, are crucial in managing NAFLD. Vitamin E should be used as an adjunct therapy to these lifestyle modifications, as it has been proven to enhance their effectiveness.

The end

www.ingramcontent.com/pod-product-compliance
Lightning Source LLC
Chambersburg PA
CBHW061320250726

48653CB00002B/977